WK 14

BEFORE THE DOCTOR COMES

A rapid reference guide to proven homoeopathic remedies for a variety of accidents, ailments and conditions, and including first-aid emergency treatments.

BEFORE THE DOCTOR COMES

by

Donovan Cox & T.W. Hyne Jones

THORSONS PUBLISHERS LIMITED
Wellingborough, Northamptonshire

Revised and Enlarged Edition 1976

ISBN 0 7225 0332 6

Filmset by Specialised Offset Services Ltd, Liverpool
Printed in Great Britain by
Weatherby Woolnough, Wellingborough
Northamptonshire

CONTENTS

PREFACE TO FIRST EDITION

This book has been written by two London businessmen who have themselves derived definite benefit from homoeopathic treatment of their own ailments after years of costly failure from ordinary medical methods. In other words, homoeopathy produces positive results and is not a whimsical theory held by a few cranks.

Arising out of their happy experiences in the use of remedies for the purposes indicated, the authors feel this information should be passed on in a simple form which can be readily understood and applied by anyone.

There is no reason why all ordinary folk should not be able to deal with quite a wide range of minor, acute troubles of their own, and of their friends needing help in this direction. Such folk will find that most homoeopathic doctors will be glad to assist and encourage them.

For those who are new to this age-old principle of healing, it may be said that all homoeopathic doctors are fully qualified physicians, but as they have graduated in homoeopathy in addition to their ordinary medical degrees, they are, in fact, 'specialists in the rational art of healing'.

The draft of this work has been submitted to various representatives of the homoeopathic profession (including two eminent London doctors) and has been approved as 'all correct and just what is wanted'.

The authors hope, therefore, that every reader will derive much benefit therefrom.

PREFACE TO REVISED, ENLARGED EDITION

It is now well over thirty years since the authors started looking for a simple and practical handbook about homoeopathy. When they could not find one, they started to write one.

The task was not so difficult as it first appeared, as all they had to do was to set down exactly what would have helped them when they began to study and to use homoeopathy. That this was the right 'yardstick' is proved by the fact that the book is still continuing to help others in a way in which they themselves would like to have been helped. The response over the years has more than fulfilled their hopes.

The reason the book has stood the test of time so well and with few alterations, is due not only to the fact that the authors were fortunate enough to be able self-administrators of the remedies, but more to the fact that homoeopathy is a true principle, a law of nature scientifically based, and consequently it is not at the mercy of whim or fashion. They have, from the outset, used and continue to use – with doctors' approval – the remedies herein described, and it is because the content of the book is just as true today as it was thirty years ago, that it was decided to publish a revised and enlarged edition.

INTRODUCTION

This book has been prepared to assist busy people to obtain relief in the case of simple accidents (such as bruises, cuts, burns and stings) and the usual run of minor domestic ailments (coughs, colds, sore throats, flu, indigestion, sickness, headaches, etc.) in the safest and simplest way – *the homoeopathic way* – without any danger of the after-effects which frequently follow the better known suppressive drugs in common use.

The information is given in such a form that it is not essential to have knowledge of homoeopathy in order to obtain some benefit from the use of these remedies.

It should, however, be understood that homoeopathy *in the fullest sense* needs a homoeopathic doctor to apply it, as every individual case needs separate individualized treatment.

However, most of the simple cases mentioned herein will readily yield to the treatment outlined in these pages. It is certain that better results can be obtained from such methods than from any other form of first-aid or domestic medicine. If the trouble is not modified or cured within a reasonable time, you should naturally exercise the common sense you would normally display and call in the doctor (preferably homoeopathic if available).

Indeed, it is by no means to replace the doctor that this book has been written, but rather to avoid wasting his time calling him to comparatively trifling cases; and at the same time to save the pockets of the general public by helping them to avoid the widely advertised chemical products which are often harmful to them in the long run. Also, apart from promoting their better health, to afford them a new field of absorbing interest.

IS HOMOEOPATHY OFFICIALLY RECOGNIZED?

Homoeopathy is widely practised in many European countries, notably in Germany and France.

The International Homoeopathic League, with a membership of 5,000, holds a congress every year, and the International Homoeopathic Research Council, with headquarters in New York, co-ordinates and sponsors research in homoeopathy throughout the world.

The clinical records of homoeopathic physicians and hospitals are evidence as to why homoeopathy is available to patients under Medicare in the United States and under the National Health Service in this country (it is also available to members of B.U.P.A.).

The Faculty of Homoeopathy is the professional body for homoeopathic doctors. It was incorporated by Act of Parliament in 1950 and part of its responsibility is for the standards of post-graduate training required by qualified practitioners. The Scottish Faculty is centred in Glasgow.

The Homoeopathic Research and Educational Trust deals with the financial side of the Faculty's educational and research work. It was established in 1948 to raise and administer funds for the advancement of the practice and teaching of homoeopathy and research.

The British Homoeopathic Association is the body working principally for laymen; it is a registered charity and was founded more than sixty years ago. Its members are men and women from all walks of life and it seeks to extend the knowledge and use of homoeopathy. The association benefits from periodic contact with the Department of Health and Social Security, Medicine Division, for mutual consultation. Membership application forms can be obtained from the Secretary. The authors strongly recommend those who are interested to become members so that they may enjoy the benefit of these facilities. Write to: The Secretary, The British Homoeopathic Association, 27a Devonshire Street, London W1N 1RJ. Tel. 01-935 2163.

There are six homoeopathic hospitals in Britain. All are in the National Health Service and provide both in-patient and out-patient facilities. They are:

The Royal London Homoeopathic Hospital, Great Ormond Street, London WC1 3HR, Tel. 01-837 3091, (out-patients) 01-837 7821.

The Glasgow Homoeopathic Hospital, 1000 Great Western Road, Glasgow W.2. Tel. 041-339 0382. (out-patients) 5 Lynedoch Crescent, Glasgow, C.3. Tel. 041-332 4490.

The Glasgow Homoeopathic Hospital for Children, 221 Hamilton Road, Glasgow E.2. Tel. 041-778 1185.

Liverpool Homoeopathic Hospital, 42 Hope Street, Liverpool L1 9DB. Tel. 051-709 8474.

The Bristol Homoeopathic Hospital, Cotham Road,

Cotham, Bristol BS6 6JU. Tel. 0272 33068, (out-patients) 0272 32007.

Tunbridge Wells Homoeopathic Hospital, Church Road, Tunbridge Wells, Kent. Tel. 0892 25065.

These are two homoeopathic clinics:

Bath Homoeopathic Clinic, Belmont, Lansdown Road, Bath. Tel. 0225 4043.

Manchester Homoeopathic Clinic, Brunswick Street, Ardwick, Manchester. Tel. 061 273 2446.

Homoeopathic Doctors

One reason for there being comparatively few homoeopathic doctors is that a doctor already qualified to practice as an M.D. needs to take an additional academic course in homoeopathy to qualify as a member of the Faculty of Homoeopathy. Therefore every homoeopathic doctor has an additional qualification and obviously the cost of achievement is much more, both in time and money.

To obtain the name, address and telephone number of your nearest homoeopathic doctor, apply to The British Homoeopathic Association, or to one of the six homoeopathic hospitals or two homoeopathic clinics in Britain. Their addresses are shown above.

WHAT IS HOMOEOPATHY?

In the Introduction it was pointed out that the information herein is given in such a form that it is not *essential* to have a knowledge of homoeopathy in order to obtain some benefit from the use of the remedies mentioned. However, it is clear that

some understanding of the principles of homoeopathy will enable anyone to use the remedies
more effectively.

The principle is, so to speak, a law of nature,
and just as an apple once dislodged from the tree
must obey a law of nature (in this case the law of
gravity) similarly homoeopathy conforms to
natural law and is, therefore, equally infallible and
unchangeable.

Homoeopathy, as a science, was established by
Samuel Hahnemann (1755-1843), an eminent
physician and chemist of Saxony. It was
introduced into England in the 1820's by Dr
Frederick Quin, physician to the Duchess of
Cambridge. In 1850 he founded the London
Homoeopathic Hospital which is today under the
patronage of Her Majesty The Queen and H.R.H.
The Duke of Gloucester.

Like Cures Like

Homoeopathy is the 'like-to-like' method in which
a particular remedy is given to the patient in small
dose, because, when given in a large dose to a
healthy person, it can produce symptoms similar
to those of the patient.

For example, if a healthy person takes a dose of
Belladonna (Deadly Nightshade), large enough to
make him ill, but *not* large enough to kill him, he
would become extremely hot, with a high
temperature, dilated pupils and a red, burning
face and throat. Therefore, according to the
homoeopathic law that *Like Cures Like*, a person
displaying such symptoms, irrespective of the
name of the disease (e.g., feverish cold of this type
or scarlet fever and so on), will be cured by

Belladonna; in fact, homoeopaths have found by experience that Belladonna is often the most useful remedy in cases of scarlet fever because the symptoms of both are so similar.

Materia Medica

However, before a substance is actually used curatively by homoeopaths, it has already been proved on a number of healthy human beings; that is to say, non-lethal doses have been taken by volunteers and all the symptoms, both mental and physical (known as 'provings') are carefully recorded and classified; these data, printed in book form, become the homoeopaths' book of reference known as the *Materia Medica*.

The approach to healing through homoeopathy is, therefore, fundamentally opposite to that of the conventional allopathic school of medicine, as, instead of attacking disease by the use of suppressive drugs, a remedy is chosen because it has been proved capable of causing similar symptoms in a healthy person. Such a remedy therefore, chosen for its similarity to the patient as a whole and not to a specific disease, activates the patient's vital or inner force and enables him to do as nature designed him to do, that is, to throw off the disease by working from within, driving the illness outwards so that it is eliminated or expelled instead of only being suppressed. The use of suppressive drugs, on the other hand, only gives temporary relief – often with unpleasant side-effects – and does not prevent the condition recurring later on.

WHAT TO BUY

Internal Remedies
(a)   Twenty-two 7g bottles of tablets or pills as follows:

Aconitum 30

ABC 30
a mixture of Aconitum
Belladonna
Chamomilla

AGE 30
a mixture of Arsenicum Iod.
Gelsemium
Eupatorium Perf.

Apis 6

Arnica 30

Arsenicum Alb. 6

Belladonna 6

Bryonia 6

Calendula 30

Cantharis 6

Carbo Veg. 6

Colocynthis 6

Gelsemium 30

Gunpowder 3x

Hypericum 30

Ignatia 30

Influenzinum-Bacillinum 30

Ipecacuanha 6

Mercurius Sol. 6

Nux Vomica 30

Pulsatilla 6

Ruta 6

Two 5 ml bottles of *Rescue Remedy* (in liquid form). This is a Dr Bach composite Flower Remedy (see page 19)

Note: The numbers following each remedy indicate the recommended potencies.

(b)   Two small bottle cases, each to hold 12 bottles.

External Remedies
(c)   Three tubes of ointment, namely:

Arnica
Calendula/Hypericum (*mixed or in separate tubes if preferred*)
Burn Ointment

(d)   One 10ml bottles of *Calendula/Hypericum* mixed tincture.

Where to Store the Remedies

Keep in a cool, dry place; away from strong light and strong-smelling substances, especially camphor, winter-green, eucalyptus, peppermint, menthol, perfume, mothballs and disinfectants.

Where to Get the Outfit

This should be bought only from homoeopathic chemists as they are specialists in handling and dispensing, and can give you good advice on the use of homoeopathic remedies.

First-aid Accessories

Cotton wool	25g pkt.
Absorbent lint	100g pkt.
2.5 and 5.0 cm W.O.W. roller bandages	3 each
Triangular bandage (useful as sling)	1
Pair of Scissors	1
Basin (to hold about 1 pint)	1
Safety pins	$\frac{1}{2}$ doz.
Eye bath	1
Medicine glass	1
$\frac{1}{2}$ min. Clinical thermometer	1

THE REMEDIES AND THEIR USE

The remedies recommended in this book are of two types – (a) for *internal* use: either tablets or pills (it does not matter which); and (b) for *external* use: ointments or tinctures. Tinctures are perhaps more effective but in certain circumstances are less easy to use and to carry than ointments.

The Dose (Internal)

A dose consists of one tablet or two pills (dissolved in the mouth) or, if in liquid form, two drops on the tongue. It should not be taken with food – preferably not after 10 min. before or not until 15 min. after. Tip the dose into the bottle cap or onto your dry hand and put straight into the mouth. Replace the cap at once.

Other medicines, aspirins, coffee and so forth, should be avoided if possible as they tend to modify or even nullify homoeopathic remedies, which are delicate and 'kindly' in their action.

Number of Doses

Generally speaking, two or three doses of the correctly chosen remedy are sufficient to relieve, modify or cure the complaint; but the golden rule is: *STOP taking the doses as soon as real improvement occurs* so that the remedy may have an opportunity to complete its action.

In other words, any number, up to about four or five doses, may be necessary to produce the desired effect. If similar symptoms return, then repeat the dose, or reconsider whether you have chosen the correct remedy. If new symptoms appear, choose the new appropriate remedy.

Certain complaints, such as colds, go through several well-defined stages, and each stage may call for a different remedy. If the symptoms continue to recur, even though alleviated from time to time, it is clear that the condition is not one for home treatment. Consult an experienced homoeopath without delay.

Frequency
Usually the more severe the attack, the shorter the interval between doses. A good general rule in these first-aid and domestic ailments is to allow half-an-hour to one hour between doses at first; lengthening the interval up to several hours after the first signs of relief occur.

How to Use the External Remedies
The ointments are easier to use for first aid purposes, and should be smeared on and preferably covered by a bandage. If using tincture, soak a dressing in solution of three drops to a tablespoonful of water, remembering that the economy of homoeopathy lies in the small quantity needed.

Compound (or Composite) Remedies
These combine two or more remedies which have been mixed together in one tablet, two or more pills, or in liquid tincture form – in other words, in one dose. This is a great help when dealing with such acute conditions as 'flu, babies' teething, accidents, agitation, etc., as speedily as possible, without recourse to aspirin (especially 'junior'), and the like. The ingredients of the remedies listed on pages 44-5 are as follows:

ABC 30 *Aconitum, Belladonna, Chamomilla*
AGE 30 *Arsenicum Iod., Gelsemium, Eupatorium Perf.*
Calendula and Hypericum *Mixed Tincture*
Rescue Remedy *Impatiens, Star of Bethlehem, Cherry Plum, Rock Rose, Clematis.*

Although Samuel Hahnemann originally prescribed single remedies for individual cases of sickness, he would, undoubtedly, have approved such suitably combined remedies for use today.

The Rescue Remedy

Associated with other remedies in this book, the *Rescue Remedy* has proved invaluable to the authors and their friends. Strictly speaking, *Rescue Remedy* is not homoeopathic, but complementary. It is a composite of the five Dr Bach Floral Remedies; *Impatiens, Star of Bethlehem, Cherry Plum, Rock Rose* and *Clematis*, which together cover 'emergency' conditions such as those after an accident while awaiting arrival of the doctor (who should be called immediately), i.e., *Before the Doctor Comes*.

Rescue will relieve shock, the effects of sudden bad news, great sorrow, a state of fear – even terror, panic and confusion. When you are awaiting some important news, about to take exams or speak in public, before going on stage, taking a driving test; whenever you are 'tensed up', bothered, 'fussed' or tired out, *Rescue* will always relieve and restore calmness and confidence, as it is a wonderful natural 'tranquillizer'. And when your mind is over-active, troubled or fearful, take a dose or two in the evening and before going to sleep.

Generally, a dose consists of 2 drops from your 5ml bottle taken, preferably, directly on the tongue, or otherwise in any drinkable liquid. If repetition is likely over, say, one or two days, put 2 drops into a 1 oz. or 20ml bottle of water and take half a teaspoonful as required.

Remember, likewise your pets and any other creatures; if they suffer fear, fright or injury, they can benefit as well from a couple of drops of *Rescue* on their food or in their drinking water.

The same principle applies in the garden and greenhouse; if you have transplanted a tree or shrub or re-potted a plant, watering and spraying with *Rescue* will counteract shock and commence rejuvenation.

Always keep a bottle of *Rescue* in the home and a small vial on your person wherever you go – you never know when you may need it suddenly, and when used, it works wonders!

Explanatory literature and advice about the Bach Flower Remedies can be obtained by sending a s.a.e. to The Secretary, The Dr Edward Bach Healing Centre, Mount Vernon, Sotwell, Wallingford, Oxon., OX10 0PZ.

ALPHABETICAL LIST OF AILMENTS

Bruises and Sprains

If the muscles or soft parts are bruised, *Arnica 30*. Apply *Arnica* Ointment (but *not* if the skin is broken, in which case use a solution of one part *Calendula-Hypericum* tincture in ten parts of warm water. For bruised bone (skull, elbow, shin bone, etc.) or strained tendons, use *Ruta 6*.

Arnica is also very useful in cases of extreme physical fatigue, say after a hard day's gardening, motoring or tennis, likewise after a long train journey, and it will combat the sort of sleeplessness that often follows over-exertion.

Should the blow be upon the fingers or toes, and especially if the spine is affected, give *Hypericum 30*.

Burns and Scalds

Quick action is necessary when severe, but keep a cool head. Shock is almost invariably involved; to control this give a dose of *Rescue Remedy at once*, and apply *Burn* Ointment. Then give a second dose of *Rescue Remedy* in five minutes' time, and a third dose in another five minutes. Give two further doses fifteen minutes apart. When shock subsides, give *Cantharis 6* to alleviate 'burning' and pain, three doses at hourly intervals. Repeat three doses if discomfort occurs, but at two-hourly intervals.

NOTE: If Burn Ointment is not available, use a *Calendula-Hypericum* dressing as prescribed for cuts, etc.

Car Exhaust or Gas Poisoning

Remove the victim at once and administer artificial respiration. Put six tablets or twelve pills of *Carbo Veg. 6* in half a teacupful of warm water, stir well and, with a small spoon, put a few drops on the tongue every ten minutes until consciousness returns, then space out the dose to every half hour.

Colds, Coughs and 'Flu

The old saying, 'prevention is better than cure', can be made more realistic by using homoeopathic remedies than by any other means. While, of course, complete immunity cannot be guaranteed, you can, more often than not, go a long way towards achieving it by taking a dose of *Influenzinum-Bacillinum 30* (or your homoeopathic chemist's own speciality) once every two weeks (if over 2 years of age).

This is a general preventive medicine, and its action is to raise one's resistance to catarrhal infections. In many cases, colds are avoided altogether; in others, the colds that are caught are less severe; they do not last so long and the unpleasant after-effects are much reduced. In some people a slight 'artificial' cold is produced, which is a good sign, indicating some toxic matter which was better out than in! Take the dose *regularly*, as prescribed above, from the beginning of October to the end of April.

If a member of the family starts a cold or influenza, all other members who have not been taking the two-weekly doses should take:

(a) Two doses of *Influenzinum-Bacillinum 30*, one on waking and the other at bedtime, but if they have already taken the two-weekly doses, then they take two doses of *AGE 30* instead. (If an influenza epidemic should break out or if one has been in contact with a person having influenza or a cold, the same procedure should be adopted).

(b) For the patient, give four doses of *AGE 30*, 2-3 hours apart, for one day. On the following day, give 3-4 doses at 3-4 hourly intervals. This compound remedy will cover most cases of colds or influenza but the following may be required in the particular circumstances described:

Aconitum 30. Chills, colds and sore throats that come on suddenly from cold, dry winds; also feverishness with quick, hard pulse. Restlessness, thirst, bursting headache, dry cough. If taken immediately symptoms appear, will often prevent development.

Arsenicum Alb. 6. Severe chills, restlessness, weakness, burning sensation. Running eyes and nose, sneezing. Loss of appetite. Shivery, thirst (if sweating) for cold drinks which relieve temporarily or for cold drinks which disagree. Gastric influenza.

Belladonna 6. Sudden chills, often after getting head wet. Flushed appearance, shining eyes, fever, throbbing frontal headache. Red, hot, dry sore throat, also nose. Tickling, dry cough, worse at night, thirsty. Cold hands and feet. In alternation with *Aconitum 30* will clear up the majority of cases which come on suddenly as the result of getting chilled.

Bryonia 6. Everything dry, worse on movement and usually by warmth. Irritable, splitting frontal headache, very thirsty. Sore throat, hard, painful cough, colds usually start in nose and travel down to chest. In alternation with *Gelsemium 30* will probably clear up seventy-five per cent of typical influenza cases.

Gelsemium 30. Great remedy for influenza colds which usually develop slowly, often in moist, mild weather. Dull, heavy, typical groggy influenza feeling, pain at back of head and at root of nose. Sneezing, sensation of lump in throat, little appetite and thirst. Dry cough, sore chest. Chilliness up and down back.

Mercurius Sol. 6. Usually indicated when the trouble has developed. Restlessness; throbbing in temples and feeling of a bandage round head. Sneezing with a greenish-yellow discharge. Putrid sore throat — often right-sided; sore gums, sometimes loss of voice. Bronchial cough with yellow expectoration. Chilly, trembling; aching bones; perspiration. Symptoms worse at night and in cold, wet weather.

Nux Vomica 30. Chills from cold dry winds. Shivery. Irritable, nervy. Stuffy nose – worse at night and outdoors. Sore throat, hoarseness, backacke, indigestion.

Pulsatilla 6. Useful for the latter stages of a cold or catarrh where there is thick yellow discharge. Nose stuffed up in the house and at night – runs in morning and outside. Wandering stitching headache. Eyes inflamed. Bad taste, not thirsty. Dry cough in evening, loose in morning. Sore chest. Often suits a mild temperament liking sympathy. Usually better out of doors.

After the patient has recovered, 3 doses of *Influenzinum-Bacillinum 30* can be taken at approximately 12-hourly intervals. This should clear up any 'hang-over' but in about three weeks it would be wise to continue the two-weekly doses as previously described.

Convulsions in Children

Convulsions in children are due to various causes such as emotional and teething troubles. If the child throws an emotional fit, call the doctor and, if possible, well moisten the baby's lips and your own with *Rescue Remedy*. Meanwhile, place the child in a warm bath, supporting the head, for 5-10 minutes, thus giving time for the fit to pass. Then dry thoroughly and wrap warmly. At the earliest opportunity repeat *Rescue Remedy* – a few further doses may be needed.

Coughs (*see* Colds)

Cuts, Grazes and Wounds

Calendula 30. One dose (together with a dose of

Rescue Remedy to deal with shock involved), may be sufficient to arrest bleeding and start the healing process – if necessary repeat in two hours.

Clean the wound, using a piece of cotton wool or unmedicated lint moistened with a solution of one part *Calendula-Hypericum* tincture in ten parts of warm water; then apply a dressing similarly moistened. Keep the solution handy in a covered tumbler. In a few hours the dressing may become dry, in which case, without removing it, moisten afresh with the solution. If it is impracticable to use a dressing, apply *Calendula* ointment after wound has been cleaned.

Dental Extractions

Take a dose of *Ignatia 30* and *Rescue Remedy* about an hour before the appointment, which will reduce the tension and fear in anticipation of the event, especially if a tooth has to be extracted. On returning home, take *Arnica 30* in alternation with *Hypericum 30* every half hour for two hours. After 24 hours, use a solution of *Calendula-Hypericum* tincture – one part in ten of warm water as a mouthwash. Repeat as necessary.

Diarrhoea

Ipecacuanha 6. Green, frothy or slimy stools. Griping around navel.

Arsenicum Alb. 6. Small, dark, offensive stools. Gnawing burning pain in abdomen. Ill effects of unripe or watery fruits and tainted food. Often much weakness. Worse late at night.

Colocynthis 6. Agonizing pain in abdomen relieved by pressure and bending double. Jelly-like stools with musty odour.

Distress (*see* Shock)

Earache
In cases of simple acute earache, the pain may be of a neuralgic type or alternatively due to a slight congestion from cold. Usually the ear should be kept warm, although occasionally warmth aggravates.

ABC 30. Often starts suddenly from chill. Some sentitivity to noises. Ears may be red and hot with acute throbbing and stabbing pains. Glands may be swollen.

Pulsatilla 6. Often follows *ABC* well. Jerking, tearing pain which usually goes through to side of the face. Ears hot and swollen. Somewhat deaf.

Mercurius Sol. 6. Pricking, tearing, pressing, burning pain often extending to cheeks. Perspiration.

In the case of children, it is especially important to call a doctor if the pain and fever do not subside quickly. This is particularly necessary if the pain is *behind* the ear, involving the mastoid bone.

Food Poisoning
Call a doctor and in the meantime give a few doses of *Arsenicum Alb. 6.*
NOTE: If the poisoning is severe, mix a dessertspoonful of mustard in a breakfastcupful of water to cause a vomit (for a child, a teaspoonful in a teacupful). After vomiting, use again the above remedy. Apply a hot compress to the stomach.

Foreign Bodies in:
(a)   *The Flesh.* If slight, these may be eased out by

gentle and equal pressure. If obstinate, a hot compress, using *Calendula-Hypericum* tincture, may be needed to soften the skin and draw out the splinter. If more severe, such as a broken needle, call a doctor. In any case, take a dose of *Hypericum 30* and *Rescue Remedy*.

(b) *The Ears*. Call a doctor. Do not syringe, or use oil drops, or thrust in a finger-tip. If agitated, take *Rescue Remedy*.

(c) *The Eyes*. *Dust*. Put a few drops of olive or castor oil under the lids. In about an hour, follow with *Calendula-Hypericum* treatment as prescribed in the following paragraph. For eyestrain from over-use, take a dose or two of *Ruta 6*.

Damaging Liquids. Put a drop of *Calendula-Hypericum* tincture in an eye-bath of warm water, tilt against the eye and open eye under water. If agitated, *Rescue Remedy*. If distress is considerable, call a doctor.

Metal Filings. Call a doctor at once, and in the meantime give two doses of *Rescue Remedy*. When the pieces have been removed, use the *Calendula-Hypericum* tincture as before – repeat as necessary.

Gas Poisoning (*see* Car Exhaust)

Grazes (*see* Cuts)

Headache
There are many causes of headaches, or it may be said there are several kinds of headaches. Like other forms of sickness, always try to determine

and remove the cause. The rightly selected homoeopathic remedy will relieve the discomfort without causing harmful after-effects, and it is far superior to the popular well-advertised remedies.

Aconitum 30. Heavy, pulsating, hot, bursting or burning. Dizzy, worse on rising. Comes on suddenly, sometimes after cold, dry wind, Often left-sided.

Arnica 30. Hot (with a cold body); confused with sharp pinching pains and a light scalp feeling. Dizzy when walking. Sometimes headache from physical fatigue or blow on head or a fall.

Belladonna 6. Particularly if due to over-exposure to sun. Hot, violent and throbbing, especially in forehead, the pain being made worse by light, noise, jar or lying down. Often right-sided, with flushed hot face.

Bryonia 6. Bursting, splitting pain in forehead, with dizziness all worse by motion.

Carbo Veg. 6. From over-eating or drinking; feels heavy and dizzy, with flatulence.

Gelsemium 30. Sometimes due to nervous anticipation. Feels heavy, as if a band around; dull, bruised, especially at back. Pain in temples. Wants a high pillow. Dizzy.

Ignatia 30. Congested, following worry, grief, or emotion, and is heavy; made worse from stooping.

Nux Vomica 30. Aches at the back or over eyes, woolly, dizzy, over-sensitive. Headache in sunshine. From over-eating and indulgence in stimulants and condiments. Often irritable.

Pulsatilla 6. Stitching pains which extend to face and teeth, often on right side. Headache from overwork. Usually applicable to the mild, emotional type. Worse from heat.

Rescue Remedy. As stress is often involved with any type of headache Rescue Remedy can usually be used to advantage in conjunction with any of the above remedies as appropriate.

Indigestion and Sickness

Arsenicum Alb. 6. Very irritable stomach and abdomen. Burning pains relieved by heat. Retching and sickness after food or drink. Sight or smell of food intolerable. Great thirst. Heartburn. Acids, ices, vegetables and water fruits disagree. Sickly appearance. Perspiration. Restlessness.

Carbo Veg. 6. Stomach and abdomen bloated, causing pain, flatulence, belching and sleepiness. Relief from passing wind, which is objectionable. Dislike of milk, meat and fats. The simplest food disagrees.

Colocynthis 6. Acute colic. Must bend double or draw legs up. Diarrhoea (like jelly) after least food or drink. Tongue rough and hot. Bitter taste. Hungry.

Gelsemium 30. Diarrhoea from emotional excitement, fright or bad news. Weakness, little appetite or thirst. Trembling.

Ignatia 30. Much flatulence. Sinking feeling. Desire for indigestible things. Diarrhoea. Troubles often caused by a fright or anger.

Ipecacuanha 6. Constant sick feeling and vomiting without relief. Clutching pain round navel. Tongue usually clean. Much saliva. Little thirst. Hiccough.

Nux Vomica 30. Biliousness due to chill. Sick feeling (worse in morning and after food) and vomiting with retching. Stomach and abdomen bloated; bruised-sore feeling, sensitive to pressure.

Weight and pain in stomach – worse some time after food. Liverish. Constipated with ineffectual urging. Ravenous hunger before a gastric attack. Fussy. Likes rich food.

Influenza (*see* Colds)

Insect Bites and Stings
Mosquito and Midge Bites. As a deterrent, wet palms of hands with a few drops of *Calendula-Hypericum* tincture and apply to hair, face, neck, wrists, ankles, etc. To allay irritation apply the tincture and take *Cantharis 6.*

Bee or Wasp Stings. Arnica 30 and *Rescue Remedy.* Apply *Burn* (or *Arnica*) ointment. Alternatively, blue-bag, or a weak solution of bi-carbonate of soda or ammonia. In fifteen minutes, *Apis 6,* followed by three more doses at hourly intervals (more frequently if sting is severe).

NOTE: If you are a beekeeper, a dose or two of *Apis 6* before going to the apiary will render stings less severe.

Horse Fly Bites. Hypericum 30 hourly, three doses. Follow with *Gunpowder 3x* three times daily for a few days. If possible, suck or squeeze the puncture immediately and then apply *Burn* (or *Arnica*) ointment.

Nettle Stings. Cantharis 6. Burn ointment.

The Monthly Period
This is frequently a time of difficulty for many young women although, as it is a natural function, it should not and need not be if the action is regularized. This is when homoeopathic remedies can be used with utmost confidence by young

women without fear of side-effects, unlike the drugs normally prescribed.

Aconitum 30. Suppressed from a fright or cold, otherwise too profuse, late and long-lasting. Vagina dry, hot, sensitive. Shooting pains. Restless.

Apis 6. Suppressed, with headache, faintness. Sensation of bearing down, tightness and tenderness. Stinging pains.

Arsenicum Alb. 6. Too early and profuse with burning pains, fatigue and better by warmth. Restless.

Belladonna 6. Too early and profuse. Bright red blood, offensive and hot. Throbbing and cutting pains.

Bryonia 6. Too early and profuse. Cutting pains, also in breasts, which are hot. Often splitting headache. Menses often preceded by nosebleed. Everything worse by motion.

Ipecacuanha 6. Too early and profuse. Blood bright red and gushing. Sickness.

Nux Vomica 30. Too early and too long-lasting. Always irregular. Blood black. Painful and constant urge to stool.

Pulsatilla 6. Too late, scanty, dark and clotted. Nervy. Pain in back and tired. Sometimes diarrhoea.

Nerves (*see* Shock)

Neuralgia

This is a painful affection of any nerve of the body. When it affects the nerves of the thigh only, it is called sciatica. The causes are many but it is generally caused by a chilling – a draught on the head, for example.

ABC 30. Sudden throbbing pain in teeth, ears, face or neck, often worse at night with hot red face and some restlessness.

Arsenicum Alb. 6. Agonizing, burning, sting, intermittent pains, usually worse after midnight, with weakness and restlessness. Better with warmth and exercise.

Colocynthis 6. Tearing pains in face and eyes – often in joints as well – aggravated by slightest touch, caused by cold and damp. Relieved by rest and warmth.

Nosebleed

Raise the arm of the side from which bleeding occurs above the head and apply something cold to the spine. Take a dose every fifteen minutes or so (two or three doses in all) of the following:

Calendula 30 in general, but *Arnica 30* if caused by a blow.

Pregnancy (calling all mothers-to-be)

During the ante-natal months, a few doses of one of the following homoeopathic remedies can help to ease many little difficulties.

Aconitum 30. Suddenness of fears. Ill effects from fears (especially of death), emotion, frights or shock. Abnormal sensitivity.

Arsenicum Alb. 6. Fussy, restless, anxious, chilly, fearful – at night. Has vomiting after meals and at night, with burning pains, thirst and diarrhoea. Better from moving about.

Ignatia 30. Nervy, sighing, anxious, frightened, sleepless, moody. Emptiness with a flat taste, distension, hiccough, retching and much lemon-coloured urine.

Ipecacuanha 6. The great nausea and morning sickness remedy when vomiting fails to relieve. Peevishness. Bleeding with bright red blood, blue rings under eyes. Usually a clean tongue.

Nux Vomica 30. Sickness, loss of appetite, constipation. Chilliness. Depression and bad temper. Longing for stimulants. Is sleepy in evening and towards morning, but sleepless in the early hours.

Pulsatilla 6. Irritability, weepiness, craving sympathy, night restlessness or vomiting of slimy matter with colic. Discoloured stools. Cracked nipples. Aversion to fats, meats, bread, milk; desire for open air. Increases expulsive power.

NOTE: As a routine measure, give a dose of *Caulophyllum 30* on Monday, Wednesday and Friday during the four weeks before baby is due. This wonderful remedy (which can be purchased additionally to those in the first-aid medicine chest), not only strengthens the particular muscles but makes them – and baby – supple. Delivery is, in consequence, easier and more natural, often obviating the need for instruments.

When the Time Comes
Unfortunately, one often hears a mother remark: 'If I have to go through all that again, I'll not have another baby' – the result of fear and pain. But, just as fortunately, when a woman has had homoeopathic remedies before and during childbirth, more often than not she declares: 'Well, if having babies is as easy as this I wouldn't mind having seven!' Just as it should be! So when the labour pains start, take a dose of *Arnica 30*

immediately; repeat in one hour, then every two hours. If things go well, probably no more than three doses in all will be necessary. *Arnica* reduces fear, shock, bruising, pain and bleeding, also risk of sepsis. After baby has arrived, take two doses of *Arnica* each day for three days.

Scalds (*see* Burns)

Septic Conditions

For all cases in which healing is slow or cuts, burns, bites, stings and so forth are inclined to fester or turn septic take, in addition to any other indicated remedy, *Gunpowder 3x* which has a strong purifying effect – three times a day for a few days, then once daily until normal, clean healing is evident.

Shock, Nerves, Distress

Aconitum 30 is a good nerve-steadier; two or three doses as required.

Arnica 30 for bruising from a fall, getting knocked or from any other physical injury and resultant shock.

Gelsemium 30 for limpness, trembling, lack of courage, exam funk or stage fright. Sensation as if stomach was turning over. For some highly-strung types this remedy has a calming effect, and covers nervous anticipation before attending a difficult interview, business meeting or other function when having to make a speech is likely.

Ignatia 30 for fright, grief from bad news; a distressed condition before a funeral or at an accident. Weeping, tendency to hysteria. For relief from emotional upset and tension.

Rescue Remedy is outstandingly a first-aid remedy in its own right and covers all the fears caused by an emergency situation; yet it is complementary to all the above and can be taken with any of them or independently.

NOTE: All the foregoing can be described as 'natural tranquillizers' without producing any side-effects and are non-habit-forming. There is a similarity between all. Choose the one you consider most suitable, but if the situation is urgent and prevents this, always use *Rescue Remedy*, which can be repeated frequently until mental relief becomes noticeable.

Sickness (*see* Indigestion)

Sleeplessness
This is usually caused either by nervous or congestive conditions such as excitement, mental activity or fear on the one hand or by indigestion on the other. Attempt to remove the cause and use one of the following remedies:

Arnica 30. Sleeplessness due to being overtired or from shock. Horrible dreams.

Nux Vomica 30. Feels drowsy in early evening; awakes in the early hours, often falling asleep just before time to get up – then feels wretched. Nervous indigestion. Irritable type.

Carbo Veg. 6. Sleeplessness probably due to lack of exercise causing indigestion. Much gas in stomach and abdomen. Often helpful to old people.

Ignatia and/or *Rescue Remedy. See under* Shock.

Sore Throat (*see* Colds)

Sprains (*see* Bruises)

Stings (*see* Insect Bites)

Teething Difficulties

Homoeopathy can save parents from many a sleepless and anxious night because of their baby, not to mention the amazing relief to the baby who is having a difficult teething time. Moreover, this relief is achieved without resorting to 'junior aspirin'.

As soon as the teething condition becomes apparent, start giving *ABC 30*. If no relief within an hour, give a second dose followed by one or two further doses at 2-3-hourly intervals if necessary. (*Rescue Remedy* can also be given in alternation or simultaneously as convenient).

This compound remedy will cover all the usual teething symptoms of restlessness, crying out through great sensitivity to pain, irritability, demand for toys which are immediately thrown down, desire to be carried, some thirst, twitching, diarrhoea. Sometimes dry cough during sleep often worse before midnight and with hot face, red on right side.

Toothache

ABC 30. Sudden throbbing pain often after exposure to cold. Teeth sensitive to cold. Gums hot and inflamed, flushed face, some restlessness.

Hypericum 30. Pain of a pulling, tearing type, made worse by cold and damp. Sensitive tooth.

Mercurius Sol. 6. Pain usually due to decay.

Wounds (*see* Cuts)

A Footnote on Diet

It should be remembered that it is natural and therefore advisable to go without food altogether for a day or two when becoming unwell, just as your dog or cat would do automatically without being taught or persuaded. Such abstinence will assist nature to hasten the action of the remedies and speed recovery. Sips of water, lemon, orange or carrot juice are usually helpful if palatable. A pure herbal laxative should be taken to keep the bowels active.

In general, health will be better maintained on a diet having a predominance of steamed and baked vegetables, dairy produce, fruit, raw salads and wholewheat bread. If there is a tendency to constipation, bran may be added with advantage. Such items as sugar, jams, sweets, pastries and cakes should be kept to a minimum as they tend to aggravate digestive troubles and contribute considerably to colds and dental decay.

Conclusion

With the help of these notes, anyone of average intelligence should be able to cope with most of the minor accidents and ailments with safety and speed, remembering that it is not necessary for *every* one of the symptoms to be present before giving the remedy.

You will soon learn by experience to differentiate between the remedies according to the main characteristics which have been given.

If you desire to become more proficient, study each medicine separately finding it in each section where it appears and noting down the symptoms given under colds, headaches, indigestion and so on. This will give you a fuller and rounder picture of the remedy as a whole.

EPIDEMICS

In addition to influenza, there are certain other acute infectious diseases which are more or less common, especially amongst children.

These have been listed along with the nosode and also the most similar homoeopathic remedies, in the form of a table (*see page 39*). The remedies printed in italics are the ones which are already in the recommended medicine chest; the remainder will need to be added if desired.

A nosode is an oral vaccine, a medicament prepared from the product of germs. It is used (on the like-to-like principle) to stimulate the body to produce natural antibodies against the particular infection.

Prevention

Judicious use of the nosodes is very helpful during an epidemic, but their greatest value is in the *prevention* of infection. For instance, if there is a case of scarlet fever at school, then let your child take *Scarlatinum 30*, one dose a week for three weeks; or if one of the children next door goes down with measles, give your own children *Morbillinum 30*, similarly. Reference to the table will show what to give in each case.

In these circumstances you would be giving what is known as a prophylactic (which one dictionary defines as treatment 'to keep guard before' or 'to ward off as in preventive treatment');

EPIDEMIC	NOSODE (Potency 30)	MOST SIMILAR REMEDIES
Chicken-pox	Varicella	Ant. Tart. 6 Rhus Tox. 6
Diphtheria	Diphtherinum	Merc. Cyan. 6
German Measles	Rubella	*Pulsatilla 6* *Belladonna 6*
Influenza	See pages 21-4	*Gelsem. 30* *Ars. Alb.* 6 *Bryonia 6*
Measles	Morbillinum	*Pulsatilla 6* *Belladonna 6*
Mumps	Parotidinum	Merc. Cor. 6 Jaborandi 3 (Pilocarpine) *Pulsatilla 6* *Belladonna 6*
Scarlet Fever	Scarlatinum	*Belladonna 6*
Smallpox	Variolinum	Ant. Tart. 6
Typhoid	Typhoidinum	*Ars. Alb.* 6 Baptisia 6 *Bryonia 6* *Merc. Sol.* 6 Pyrogen 30 Rhus Tox. 6
Whooping Cough	Pertussin (Coqueluchin)	Drosera 6

this will either prevent an attack developing or, if one does develop, it will render it less severe by reducing predisposition; for, as Dr Alfred Pulford has pointed out, 'No disease will arise without an existing predisposition to any particular disease that makes us immune to it. Homoeopathy alone is capable of removing these predispositions.

Treatment
If symptoms start developing, use in addition the best of the most similar remedies, and notify the doctor immediately.

After-Effects
In cases which were not treated homoeopathically at the time, after-effects (or as the doctors would say, 'sequelae'), may develop. It matters little what form these sequelae take; it may be ear trouble, it may be rheumatism, it may be kidney trouble or just a 'never-very-well-feeling'; the appropriate nosode, according to the original trouble, will work wonders. Give 3 doses (bed-time, on waking, bed-time). There may be some slight reaction during the ensuing 10 days. If so, take another 3 doses 2 weeks later. If the trouble is a true after-effect from the improperly treated original infection, you can feel confident of improvement, even if the origin was several years ago.

Vaccination and Injections
Although we dislike these in principle, they are inevitable in these days of constant world travel in order to comply with official regulations. We recommend, however, that a homoeopathic physician be consulted.

SOME QUESTIONS ANSWERED

Can Homoeopathy Fail?

From the foregoing, it may be asked if it is possible for there ever to be a failure? Indeed, it is not, provided that the patient is not beyond cure and the medicine given in minute quantities is similar (homoeopathic) to the patient and would therefore cause similar illness symptoms if given in large doses to a healthy person.

Unfortunately, however, human nature is apt to err sometimes; for example, the patient may unwittingly fail to give a complete and accurate account of his symptoms, or may even deliberately suppress some important fact. In this event, there may be temporary failure, necessitating a review of the case.

Fortunately, the dose used is so infinitesimal that, as experience has shown for over 150 years, *provided it is not repeated over too long a period*, it will do no harm even when it fails; the failure being due to *the dose not being homoeopathic (or similar)*.

It will be seen, therefore, that the patient should always endeavour to give the doctor the fullest information, so that improvement and success may be achieved as soon as possible.

Remember, the like-to-like law is infallible, but it is in our efforts to apply the law that failure may occur, so that in the few cases where there is failure, it is *we* who fail – not homoeopathy.

What Is a 'Potency'?

When he made his first experiments, over 150 years ago, Dr Samuel Hahnemann found that large and frequent doses of the 'similar', although usually an effective cure in the long run, often caused an aggravation of the patient's condition before the cure was complete. This revealed the important the fact that the smaller the dose, the greater the power. Present-day atomic scientists have discovered the same fact and, by finer sub-division of the original element have produced greater and greater power. In homoeopathy, these finer sub-divisions are produced by progressive, predetermined dilution and succussion (vigorous shaking) until the required potency has been obtained.

One advantage of the very small dose, from the patient's point of view, is that is leaves no harmful after-effects, which is more than can be said for the increasing number of powerful drugs in common use.

So we see that homoeopathy, through the application of the 'minimum' dose of the 'similar' remedy (or 'similimum'), gently stimulates the vital force so as to set in action the patient's own healing process from the centre of his being, working steadily outwards until the disease is totally expelled and harmony is restored.

Is There a Homoeopathic Tonic?

All homoeopathic remedies, being directed towards healing the whole person, are tonics in themselves. However, after acute illnesses such as influenza or during a pregnancy and other anaemic conditions for which iron therapy might otherwise be prescribed, a compound of *Calc. Phos. 3x* and *Ferr. Phos. 2x* is often highly beneficial.

Is Homoeopathy a Form of Herbalism?

No. Homoeopathy makes use of most substances, vegetable and mineral, and it is based not so much on a particular class of remedy as in herbalism, but in the specialized way the remedies are selected, prepared and prescribed.

Is Aspirin Harmful?

It is well known that neither doctors nor manufacturing chemists claim that aspirin or aspirin-based compounds actually *cure*; they do no more than alleviate. In a 1973 television programme it was pointed out that aspirin (and many other drugs) cause some stomach haemorrhage. Naturally, the amount of internal bleeding varies from person to person but, if the use of aspirin is persisted in, it can be very harmful, for example, in cases of stomach ulcers.

According to a report in a leading medical journal, chronic aspirin ingestion in children is not uncommon; it often goes undetected and may cause serious anaemia from blood loss. Unfortunately, parents do not seem to consider aspirin as a drug and they give it to their children as a pain-reliever or sedative without a second thought. One of the cases in the study, involved an eight-month-old infant who had been given 'junior aspirin' to relieve teething pains for six weeks running. The other children in the family had all received aspirin regularly for a period of between six weeks and six months. They all developed anaemia, the main symptoms being listlessness and pallor. The treatment that the doctors found effective was discontinuance of the aspirin, followed by iron therapy.

INDEX OF REMEDIES

ABC 30. Babies' teething, toothache, earache, etc.

Aconitum 30. Agitation, shock, chills, colds, coughs, sore throats, headaches, neuralgia, earache, toothache, pregnancy, monthly period.

AGE 30. Colds, 'flu, sore throats, coughs.

Apis 6. Bee and wasp stings, headache, monthly period.

Arnica 30. Bruises, fatigue, sleeplessness, physical shock, blows, stings, dental extraction, falls, nosebleed, headache, childbirth.

Arsenicum Album 6. Colds, chills, 'flu, cough, indigestion, sickness, diarrhoea, neuralgia, pregnancy, monthly period, typhoid.

Belladonna 6. Chills, sore throat, cough, headache, neuralgia, earache, toothache, gumboils, teething, convulsions, monthly period, scarlet fever, measles, mumps.

Bryonia 6. Cough, 'flu, sore throat, colds, indigestion and sickness, headaches, monthly period.

Calendula 30. Cuts, wounds, grazes, nosebleeds.

Cantharis 6. Burns and scalds, mosquito and midge bites, nettle stings.

Carbo Vegetabilis 6. Food poisoning, car exhaust or coal gas poisoning, indigestion and sickness, headache.

Colocynthis 6. Indigestion and sickness, diarrhoea, neuralgia.

Gelsemium 30. Shock, 'flu, colds, chills, coughs, sore throat, headache, indigestion and sickness.

Gunpowder 3x. Horse-fly bites, septic conditions, slow healing, festering, blood-purifier.

Hypericum 30. Acutely painful cuts, wounds, grazes, blows on fingers or toes or especially spine, foreign bodies in flesh, horse-fly bites, toothache before dental extraction or filling.

Ignatia 30. Agitation, nervous shock, indigestion and sickness, headache, convulsions, pregnancy.

Influenzinum-Bacillinum 30. General preventive against colds, 'flu, etc., and to clear up after effects.

Ipecacuanha 6. Sickness and nausea, diarrhoea, pregnancy, monthly period.

Mercurius Solubilus 6. 'Flu, chills, colds, cough, sore throat, diarrhoea, headache, earache, toothache, gum troubles, typhoid.

Nux Vomica 30. Chills, sore throat, colds, indigestion and sickness, headache, convulsions, pregnancy, monthly period.

Pulsatilla 6. Colds, catarrh, cough, sore throat, measles, indigestion and sickness, headache, earache, pregnancy, monthly period, mumps.

Rescue Remedy. Shock, fear, terror, panic, confusion, 'stage-nerves', exhaustion, or any emergency situation.

Ruta 6. Bruised bone, strained tendons, eye strain.

INDEX